THE ULTIMATE GUIDE TO NUTRIRITON AND FITNESS FOR ALL AGES

A.C. Stallings RN

independent

ISBN-13: 9798393006549

Cover design by: Art Painter
Library of Congress Control Number: 2018675309
Printed in the United States of America

*This book is dedicated to my family and
friends who encourage me to write.*

"To eat is a necessity, but to eat intelligently is an art"

LA ROCHEFOUCAULD

CONTENTS

INTRODUCTION

Nutrition and fitness are two vital components of a healthy lifestyle. They are interconnected and work together to help you achieve your health goals. This guide will provide you with invaluable insight into good nutrition that provides your body with necessary nutrients to function properly, and how regular exercise assists in keeping your body in shape and improving overall health.

PREFACE

Staying healthy is important, no matter your age. Good nutrition and fitness are crucial for maintaining a healthy body. A balanced diet filled with fruits, vegetables, whole grains, lean proteins, and healthy fats provides your body with essential nutrients to help it thrive. Engage in regular exercise to keep your muscles and bones strong, improve cardiovascular health, and boost energy. Strength training, cardio, or yoga – whatever your preferred exercise routine may be – it all counts.

INTRODUCTION

Why nutrition and fitness matter

Why Nutrition and Fitness Matter

Nutrition and fitness are two essential components of a healthy lifestyle. They are interconnected and work together to help you achieve your health goals. Good nutrition provides your body with the necessary nutrients to function properly, while regular exercise helps keep your body in shape and improves overall health.

Nutrition and Fitness for All Ages

Regardless of your age, good nutrition and fitness are crucial for maintaining good health. Eating a balanced diet that includes plenty of fruits, vegetables, whole grains, lean proteins, and healthy fats is essential for providing your body with the nutrients it needs to thrive. Regular exercise is equally important, whether it's through strength training, cardio, or yoga. Exercise helps keep your muscles and bones strong, improves cardiovascular health, and boosts energy levels.

Plant-Based Nutrition and Fitness

Plant-based nutrition and fitness is becoming increasingly popular as more people are embracing a vegan or vegetarian lifestyle. A plant-based diet can provide all the necessary nutrients for good health, including protein, iron, calcium, and vitamins. Plant-based fitness can include activities like hiking, biking, and yoga, among others. Eating a plant-based diet and engaging in regular physical activity can help reduce the risk of chronic diseases like obesity, diabetes, and heart disease.

Holistic Nutrition and Fitness

Holistic nutrition and fitness focus on the whole person, including physical, mental, and emotional health. This approach emphasizes the importance of a balanced diet, regular exercise, stress management, and self-care practices like meditation and mindfulness. Holistic nutrition and fitness can help improve overall health and well-being by addressing the root causes of health issues.

Weight Loss Nutrition and Fitness

Losing weight requires a combination of good nutrition and regular exercise. A healthy diet that includes plenty of fruits, vegetables, lean proteins, and whole grains can help you lose weight and maintain a healthy weight. Regular exercise, such as strength training and cardio, can help burn calories, increase metabolism, and build muscle mass.

Nutrition and Fitness for Seniors

As we age, good nutrition and fitness become even more important. Eating a balanced diet that includes plenty of fruits, vegetables, lean proteins, and whole grains can help prevent chronic diseases and maintain cognitive function. Regular exercise, such as walking, swimming, or yoga, can help maintain muscle mass, improve balance, and reduce the risk of falls.

Nutrition and Fitness for Children

Good nutrition and fitness habits should start early in life. A balanced diet that includes plenty of fruits, vegetables, whole grains, lean proteins, and healthy fats is essential for children's growth and development. Regular physical activity is also important for building strong bones and muscles and improving cardiovascular health.

Nutrition and Fitness for Busy Professionals

Even if you have a busy schedule, it's important to make time for good nutrition and fitness. Meal planning, meal prep, and packing healthy snacks can help you maintain a healthy diet, even when you're on the go. Regular exercise, such as high-intensity interval training (HIIT), can help you stay in shape and boost energy levels, even when you don't have a lot of time.

In conclusion, good nutrition and fitness are essential for maintaining good health at any age. Eating a balanced diet and engaging in regular physical activity can help prevent chronic diseases, maintain a healthy weight, and improve overall well-being. Whether you're interested in plant-based nutrition and fitness, holistic nutrition and fitness, weight loss nutrition and fitness, or nutrition and fitness for seniors, children, or busy professionals, there are plenty of options available to help you achieve your health goals.

The benefits of a healthy lifestyle

Living a healthy lifestyle is essential for everyone, regardless of age or occupation. A healthy lifestyle is a combination of good nutrition and regular exercise, and it has numerous benefits. Here are some of the benefits of a healthy lifestyle:

1. Improved Physical Health

Eating a balanced diet and engaging in regular exercise can help you maintain a healthy weight, reduce the risk of chronic diseases like diabetes, heart disease, and cancer, and boost your overall physical health. A healthy lifestyle can also improve your immune system, making you less susceptible to illnesses.

2. Mental Health Benefits

Maintaining a healthy lifestyle has numerous mental health benefits, including reducing stress and anxiety, improving mood, and boosting self-esteem. Exercise releases endorphins, which are natural mood boosters, and eating a healthy diet can also have a positive impact on mental health.

3. Increased Energy Levels

Eating a healthy diet and engaging in regular exercise can boost energy levels, making it easier to get through the day without feeling fatigued. This is particularly beneficial for busy professionals who need to be alert and focused throughout the day.

4. Improved Sleep

A healthy lifestyle can also improve the quality of sleep, helping you wake up feeling refreshed and energized. Exercise can help regulate sleep patterns, while a balanced diet can reduce sleep disturbances.

5. Longevity

Living a healthy lifestyle can increase your lifespan, allowing you to enjoy a longer, healthier life. Seniors, in particular, can benefit from a healthy lifestyle, as it can help them maintain their independence and quality of life.

6. Weight Loss

A healthy lifestyle can also help with weight loss, particularly when combined with a calorie-controlled diet. Plant-based nutrition and fitness, in particular, can be effective for weight loss, as plant-based foods tend to be lower in calories and higher in fiber.

7. Improved Cognitive Function

Eating a healthy diet and engaging in regular exercise can also improve cognitive function, including memory, concentration, and focus. This is particularly beneficial for children, as it can help them perform better in school.

In conclusion, a healthy lifestyle has numerous benefits, including improved physical and mental health, increased energy levels, improved sleep, longevity, weight loss, and improved cognitive function. Regardless of your age or occupation, it's never too late to start living a healthy lifestyle.

The importance of nutrition and fitness for all ages

Nutrition and fitness are essential for everyone, regardless of age or lifestyle. They play a critical role in maintaining optimal health and preventing chronic diseases. A well-balanced diet combined with regular physical activity can help individuals achieve and maintain a healthy weight, improve mental health, boost energy levels, and reduce the risk of a variety of health problems.

For individuals who follow a plant-based diet, it is essential to ensure they are getting all the necessary nutrients. Plant-based protein sources such as beans, lentils, and nuts can help meet the body's protein needs. Additionally, consuming a variety of fruits, vegetables, whole grains, and healthy fats can provide the necessary vitamins, minerals, and antioxidants to support overall health.

Holistic nutrition and fitness focus on the connection between the mind, body, and spirit. It involves incorporating healthy habits such as mindfulness, meditation, and stress-management techniques into one's lifestyle. This approach can help individuals achieve a healthy balance and promote optimal health.

Weight loss nutrition and fitness are essential for individuals looking to lose weight and improve their overall health. A calorie-controlled diet, combined with regular physical activity, can help individuals achieve their weight loss goals. It is also important to focus on consuming nutrient-dense foods and limiting processed and high-calorie foods.

As individuals age, their nutritional needs may change. Nutrition and fitness for seniors can help meet these changing needs. Adequate protein, calcium, and vitamin D are essential to maintaining bone health, while consuming a variety of fruits, vegetables, and whole grains can help support overall health.

Nutrition and fitness for children are critical for promoting healthy growth and development. It is essential to provide children with a well-balanced diet that includes plenty of fruits, vegetables, whole grains, and lean protein sources. Regular physical activity can also help promote a healthy weight, improve mental health, and support healthy growth and development.

Nutrition and fitness for busy professionals can be challenging but are essential for maintaining optimal health. Planning meals and snacks in advance and scheduling regular physical activity can help busy individuals stay on track with their health goals.

In conclusion, nutrition and fitness are essential for all ages and lifestyles. By incorporating healthy habits into one's lifestyle, individuals can achieve and maintain optimal health, prevent chronic diseases, and improve overall well-being.

Nutrition and Fitness Basics

The Basics Of Nutrition

The basics of nutrition are essential for leading a healthy and active lifestyle. Nutrition is the process of providing the body with the necessary nutrients and energy to function correctly. There are six essential nutrients that the body requires: carbohydrates, proteins, fats, vitamins, minerals, and water.

Carbohydrates are the primary energy source for the body. They are found in grains, fruits, vegetables, and dairy products. Proteins are necessary for building and repairing tissues, and they can be found in animal products such as meat, fish, and eggs, as well as plant-based sources such as beans and nuts. Fats are essential for hormone production and cell function and can be found in oils, nuts, and seeds.

Vitamins and minerals are essential for various bodily functions, including bone health, immune function, and energy production. These nutrients can be found in a variety of foods, including fruits, vegetables, whole grains, and dairy products. Water is vital for hydration and helps regulate body temperature.

It is essential to maintain a balanced diet that includes a variety of nutrient-dense foods. A balanced diet should include a mix of carbohydrates, proteins, and fats, along with plenty of fruits and vegetables. It is also important to limit processed foods and foods high in sugar and saturated fats.

Incorporating physical activity into your daily routine is also essential for overall health and wellness. Exercise can help reduce the risk of chronic diseases, improve mood, and increase energy levels. Aim for at least 150 minutes of moderate-intensity exercise per week, such as brisk walking, cycling, or swimming.

Different age groups have different nutritional needs. Seniors may require more calcium and vitamin D to maintain bone health, while children need more protein and calcium for growth and development. Busy professionals may benefit from meal prepping and planning to ensure they are getting the necessary nutrients during their hectic schedules.

In conclusion, the basics of nutrition include a balanced diet that includes carbohydrates, proteins, fats, vitamins, minerals, and water. It is also important to incorporate physical activity into your daily routine and tailor your nutritional needs based on your age and lifestyle. By following these simple guidelines, you can lead a healthy and active lifestyle for all ages.

Macronutrients

Macronutrients are essential nutrients required in large amounts by the body to provide energy and support growth and development. They include carbohydrates, proteins, and fats and are found in a variety of foods.

Carbohydrates are the primary source of energy for the body. They are found in foods such as fruits, vegetables, grains, and dairy products. Carbohydrates are broken down into glucose, which is used by the body as fuel. It is important to consume complex carbohydrates, such as whole grains, as they provide more sustained energy compared to simple carbohydrates found in sugary foods.

Proteins are essential for building and repairing tissues and for the production of enzymes and hormones. They are found in foods such as meat, poultry, fish, beans, and nuts. It is important to consume a variety of protein sources to ensure adequate intake of all essential amino acids.

Fats are essential for the absorption of vitamins and minerals and for the production of hormones. They are found in foods such as avocados, nuts, seeds, and oils. It is important to consume healthy fats, such as monounsaturated and polyunsaturated fats while limiting saturated and trans fats.

It is important to consume an appropriate balance of macronutrients to promote overall health and wellness. A balanced diet should consist of approximately 50% carbohydrates, 20% proteins, and 30% fats. However, individual needs may vary based on factors such as age, gender, and physical activity level.

For those following a plant-based diet, it is important to consume a variety of plant-based protein sources, such as legumes, tofu, and tempeh, to ensure adequate protein intake. It is also important to incorporate healthy plant-based fats, such as those found in nuts and seeds, into the diet.

For those focused on weight loss, it is important to consume a calorie-controlled diet that still includes all macronutrients. It is also important to focus on consuming whole, nutrient-dense foods rather than highly processed foods.

For seniors and children, it is important to ensure adequate intake of all macronutrients to support growth, development, and overall health. It may also be necessary to adjust macronutrient intake based on individual needs and medical conditions.

For busy professionals, meal planning and preparation can help ensure a balanced diet that includes all macronutrients. It is also important to choose convenient, healthy food options when eating out or on the go.

In summary, macronutrients are essential for overall health and wellness. It is important to consume a balanced diet that includes all macronutrients in appropriate amounts to support energy, growth, and development. Individual needs may vary based on factors such as age, gender, and physical activity level.

Micronutrients

Micronutrients are essential nutrients that the body requires in small amounts to maintain proper functioning. These include vitamins, minerals, and trace elements. Although they are needed in small quantities, they play a significant role in maintaining good health and preventing diseases.

Vitamins are organic compounds that are required in small quantities for various metabolic processes in the body. They are essential for maintaining healthy skin, bones, and teeth, and are essential for the proper functioning of the immune system. Vitamins are divided into two categories: water-soluble and fat-soluble. Water-soluble vitamins include vitamin C and the B-complex vitamins, while fat-soluble vitamins include vitamins A, D, E, and K.

Minerals are inorganic substances that are required in small quantities for various functions in the body. They are essential for maintaining healthy bones, teeth, and muscles, as well as for the proper functioning of the nervous system. Minerals are classified into two categories: major minerals and trace minerals. Major minerals include calcium, magnesium, and potassium, while trace minerals include iron, zinc, and selenium.

Trace elements are essential micronutrients that are required in very small quantities for various metabolic processes in the body. They are important for the proper functioning of enzymes and proteins, as well as for the maintenance of healthy bones, teeth, and muscles. Trace elements include copper, iodine, and manganese.

Micronutrient deficiencies can lead to a wide range of health problems, including anemia, osteoporosis, and immune system dysfunction. It is important to consume a well-balanced diet that includes a variety of fruits, vegetables, whole grains, lean proteins, and healthy fats to ensure that you are getting all the micronutrients your body needs.

In conclusion, micronutrients play a vital role in maintaining good health and preventing diseases. It is important to consume a well-balanced diet that includes a variety of fruits, vegetables, whole grains, lean proteins, and healthy fats to ensure that you are getting all the micronutrients your body needs. If you are unable to get enough micronutrients from your diet alone, you may need to consider taking supplements under the guidance of a healthcare professional.

Water

Water is an essential nutrient that is necessary for life. It makes up about 60% of our body weight and is involved in many bodily functions such as regulating body temperature, transporting nutrients, and flushing out waste products. It is important to stay hydrated throughout the day to maintain optimal health and performance.

For individuals who are pursuing a plant-based nutrition and fitness lifestyle, it is important to note that many plant-based foods have a high water content, such as fruits and vegetables. This can help maintain hydration levels.

Holistic nutrition and fitness advocates for drinking water that is free from contaminants, such as chemicals and heavy metals. It is recommended to drink filtered or purified water to reduce exposure to these harmful substances.

For those who are looking to lose weight, drinking water can be a helpful tool. Drinking water before meals can help reduce appetite and lead to consuming fewer calories overall. Additionally, staying hydrated can help reduce water retention and bloating.

Seniors and children both have unique hydration needs. Seniors may have reduced thirst sensations and may need to consciously make an effort to drink water throughout the day. Children may need reminders to drink water, especially during physical activity or in hot weather.

For busy professionals, it can be easy to forget to drink enough water during the day. Keeping a water bottle nearby and setting reminders can help ensure adequate hydration.

In summary, water is an essential nutrient that is necessary for optimal health and performance. It is important to stay hydrated throughout the day, especially for those pursuing plant-based, holistic, weight loss, senior, and children's nutrition and fitness lifestyles. Busy professionals can benefit from setting reminders and keeping a water bottle nearby. Remember to prioritize hydration for overall health and wellness.

The Basics Of Fitness

The Basics of Fitness

Fitness is a critical component of a healthy lifestyle. It is essential to maintain good physical and mental health, and it has numerous benefits that can enhance your quality of life. Whether you are a beginner or a seasoned fitness enthusiast, it is important to learn the basics of fitness to achieve your fitness goals.

The first step towards achieving fitness is to understand the components of fitness. Fitness consists of several components, including cardiovascular endurance, muscular strength, muscular endurance, flexibility, and body composition. Each of these components plays a significant role in improving your overall fitness.

Cardiovascular endurance refers to the ability of your heart, lungs and circulatory system to deliver oxygen and nutrients to your muscles during exercise. It is essential for activities that involve sustained physical activity, such as running, swimming, or cycling.

Muscular strength is the ability of your muscles to generate force against resistance. It is important for activities that require lifting or pushing, such as weightlifting or pushing a heavy object.

Muscular endurance is the ability of your muscles to perform repeated contractions without fatigue. It is essential for activities that require sustained physical effort, such as running a marathon or performing multiple repetitions of an exercise.

Flexibility refers to the range of motion of your joints and muscles. It is important for activities that require a wide range of motion, such as gymnastics or dancing.

Body composition refers to the proportion of fat, muscle, and bone in your body. It is important for overall health, as excessive body fat can increase the risk of chronic diseases such as heart disease and diabetes.

To improve your fitness, you need to engage in regular physical activity that targets each of these components. This can include a combination of cardiovascular exercise, strength training, and flexibility exercises.

Cardiovascular exercise can include activities such as running, cycling, swimming, or brisk walking. Aim for at least 150 minutes of moderate-intensity cardiovascular exercise per week.

Strength training can include exercises such as weightlifting, bodyweight exercises, or resistance band exercises. Aim for at least two strength training sessions per week, targeting all major muscle groups.

Flexibility exercises can include stretching, yoga, or Pilates. Aim for at least two flexibility sessions per week.

In addition to regular physical activity, it is essential to maintain a healthy diet to support your fitness goals. A balanced diet that includes plenty of fruits, vegetables, whole grains, lean protein, and healthy fats can provide the nutrients your body needs to perform at its best.

In conclusion, fitness is a critical component of a healthy lifestyle that can offer numerous benefits for individuals of all ages. Understanding the basics of fitness and engaging in regular physical activity and a healthy diet can help you achieve your fitness goals and improve your overall health and well-being.

Cardiovascular Exercise

Cardiovascular exercise is a type of physical activity that is designed to increase heart rate and blood flow throughout the body. It is one of the most important forms of exercise for overall health and fitness, and it can be done in a variety of ways.

Cardiovascular exercise can be done through activities such as running, cycling, swimming, dancing, and even walking. It can be done indoors or outdoors, and can be done alone or with a group of people.

The benefits of cardiovascular exercise are numerous. It can help to improve heart health, increase lung capacity, reduce the risk of chronic diseases such as diabetes and heart disease, improve mental health, and even aid in weight loss. Additionally, it can help to improve overall physical fitness and stamina, making it easier to perform daily activities and enjoy life to the fullest.

For those interested in plant-based nutrition and fitness, there are many options for cardiovascular exercise. Activities such as hiking, rock climbing, and yoga can be great ways to get the heart pumping while also connecting with nature and the environment. For those interested in holistic nutrition and fitness, activities such as tai chi and qigong can be great ways to improve overall health and well-being while also getting the heart pumping.

For those interested in weight loss nutrition and fitness, cardiovascular exercise can be an essential component of a successful weight loss plan. Increasing heart rate and burning calories, it can help to create a calorie deficit and promote weight loss over time.

For seniors, children, and busy professionals, cardiovascular exercise can be tailored to meet specific needs and preferences. For seniors, low-impact activities such as walking and gentle yoga can be great options. For children, activities such as sports and games can be fun ways to get the heart pumping. And for busy professionals, activities such as short bursts of high-intensity interval training (HIIT) can be great ways to fit in a quick workout during a busy day.

Overall, cardiovascular exercise is an important aspect of overall health and fitness for all ages and niches. By incorporating it into a balanced nutrition and fitness plan, individuals can reap the many benefits of improved heart health, increased stamina, and overall well-being.

Strength Training

Strength training is an essential part of any fitness routine, no matter your age or fitness level. It involves exercises that target your muscles, bones, and connective tissues, helping to improve your overall strength, balance, and coordination. Not only can strength training help you to build muscle and improve your physical performance, but it can also have numerous health benefits, including reducing the risk of chronic disease, improving bone density, and increasing metabolism.

One of the biggest misconceptions about strength training is that it is only for bodybuilders or athletes. However, strength training can be beneficial for people of all ages and fitness levels, including seniors and children. For seniors, strength training can help to improve balance and prevent falls, while for children, it can help to build strong bones and muscles and improve overall physical fitness.

When it comes to strength training, there are a few key principles to keep in mind. First, it is important to start with a weight that is challenging but manageable for you. This will help you to build strength and avoid injury. Additionally, it is important to vary your exercises and routines to target different muscle groups and prevent boredom.

For those following a plant-based or holistic diet, strength training can still be a great addition to your fitness routine. Plant-based protein sources such as beans, lentils, and tofu can provide the necessary nutrients for muscle growth and repair, while holistic practices such as yoga and Pilates can help to improve flexibility and balance.

For those looking to lose weight, strength training can also be a valuable tool. Building muscle can help to increase metabolism and burn more calories, even at rest. Additionally, strength training can help to tone and shape your body, improving overall body composition.

Finally, for busy professionals, strength training can be a great way to incorporate exercise into a busy schedule. Short, intense workouts can be just as effective as longer workouts and can be done in the comfort of your own home or at a gym.

Overall, strength training is an important part of any fitness routine, providing numerous benefits for people of all ages and fitness levels. Whether you are looking to build muscle, lose weight, or improve your overall health and fitness, incorporating strength training into your routine can help you to achieve your goals.

Flexibility training

Flexibility training is an essential component of any fitness routine, regardless of age or fitness level. It involves stretching and lengthening muscles to improve the range of motion, reduce the risk of injury, and enhance athletic performance.

There are several types of flexibility training, including static stretching, dynamic stretching, and proprioceptive neuromuscular facilitation (PNF). Static stretching involves holding a stretch for a certain period of time, while dynamic stretching involves moving through a range of motion. PNF combines both static and dynamic stretching, along with muscle contractions, to improve flexibility.

Flexibility training can be especially beneficial for seniors, as it can help maintain mobility and prevent falls. It can also benefit children by improving their posture and coordination. Busy professionals can benefit from flexibility training as well, as it can help reduce stress and tension in the body.

Plant-based nutrition and fitness enthusiasts can use flexibility training to complement their workouts, as it can help prevent muscle imbalances and injury. Holistic nutrition and fitness practitioners can use flexibility training as part of a well-rounded approach to health and wellness.

Regardless of your fitness goals, incorporating flexibility training into your routine can help improve your overall fitness and well-being. It is important to remember to warm up before stretching and to hold stretches for at least 30 seconds to allow the muscle to fully lengthen.

In conclusion, flexibility training is an important aspect of any fitness routine and can benefit individuals of all ages and fitness levels. Whether you are looking to improve athletic performance, prevent injury, or simply maintain mobility, incorporating flexibility training into your routine can help you achieve your goals.

PLANT-BASED NUTRITION AND FITNESS

What is plant-based nutrition?

Plant-based nutrition is a dietary approach that emphasizes the consumption of whole foods derived from plants such as fruits, vegetables, grains, legumes, nuts, and seeds. Unlike the conventional Western diet that is high in processed and animal-based foods, plant-based nutrition is centered around nutrient-dense, fiber-rich, and low-calorie foods that offer a wide range of health benefits.

Plant-based nutrition has gained popularity in recent years due to its potential to improve health outcomes and reduce the risk of chronic diseases such as heart disease, diabetes, and cancer. Numerous studies have demonstrated the benefits of plant-based diets in promoting weight loss, improving blood sugar control, reducing inflammation, and enhancing overall well-being.

A plant-based diet is not necessarily a vegan or vegetarian diet, although these diets fall within the plant-based spectrum. It is possible to follow a plant-based diet while still consuming some animal products, albeit in smaller quantities and less frequently. The key is to prioritize plant-based foods as the foundation of your diet and to limit or eliminate processed and animal-based foods.

Adopting a plant-based diet may seem daunting, especially for those who are used to a diet rich in meat and dairy products. However, the transition can be gradual and personalized to fit your preferences and lifestyle. Here are some tips to get started with plant-based nutrition:

1. Start by incorporating more plant-based foods into your meals. This could mean adding more fruits and vegetables to your plate, swapping meat for legumes or tofu, or using nut milk instead of dairy milk.

2. Experiment with different plant-based recipes and cuisines. There are countless delicious and nutritious plant-based dishes that can cater to different tastes and preferences.

3. Pay attention to nutrient balance and variety. Make sure you are getting enough protein, healthy fats, and essential micronutrients by including a variety of plant-based foods in your diet.

4. Don't forget about physical activity. Plant-based nutrition is only one aspect of a healthy lifestyle. Regular exercise and physical activity are essential for optimal health and well-being.

In summary, plant-based nutrition is a dietary approach that emphasizes the consumption of whole foods derived from plants. It offers numerous health benefits and can be personalized to fit different lifestyles and preferences. By adopting a plant-based diet, you can improve your health outcomes, reduce the risk of chronic diseases, and enhance your overall well-being.

Benefits Of A Plant-Based Diet

A plant-based diet consists of foods that are derived from plants such as fruits, vegetables, whole grains, legumes, nuts, and seeds. It is a way of eating that emphasizes whole, minimally processed foods while limiting or eliminating animal products. There are numerous benefits of following a plant-based diet, and here are some of them:

1. Improved heart health: A plant-based diet can help reduce the risk of heart disease by lowering blood pressure, reducing cholesterol levels, and preventing the formation of blood clots.

2. Better weight management: Plant-based diets are typically lower in calories and higher in fiber, which can help you feel fuller for longer and promote weight loss.

3. Reduced risk of cancer: Research has shown that plant-based diets may reduce the risk of certain types of cancer, including breast, colon, and prostate cancer.

4. Improved digestion: Plant-based diets are rich in fiber, which can help regulate digestion and prevent constipation.

5. Increased energy: Plant-based diets are typically rich in vitamins, minerals, and antioxidants, which can help boost energy levels and improve overall health.

6. Better brain function: Plant-based diets are rich in nutrients that are important for brain health, such as omega-3 fatty acids, B vitamins, and antioxidants.

7. Reduced inflammation: Plant-based diets are naturally anti-inflammatory, which can help reduce the risk of chronic diseases such as arthritis and diabetes.

8. Improved immune function: Plant-based diets are rich in nutrients that are important for immune function, such as vitamin C, vitamin E, and zinc.

9. Better environmental sustainability: Plant-based diets have a lower environmental impact than diets that include animal products, as they require fewer resources to produce.

Overall, a plant-based diet can be a healthy and sustainable way of eating for all ages and all niches of nutrition and fitness. Whether you are looking to improve your heart health, manage your weight, or reduce your risk of chronic disease, a plant-based diet can be a great option.

How To Transition To A Plant-Based Diet

Transitioning to a plant-based diet can be a daunting task, especially if you are used to consuming meat and dairy products regularly. However, with the right mindset and approach, it can be a rewarding and healthy lifestyle change that can benefit your overall health and well-being. Here are some tips on how to transition to a plant-based diet:

1. Start Slowly

It is essential to take your time when transitioning to a plant-based diet. Start by incorporating one plant-based meal into your daily routine and gradually increase the number of plant-based meals until you are fully comfortable with the lifestyle.

2. Educate Yourself

Research on plant-based nutrition to understand the benefits, the types of foods that provide the necessary nutrients, and the potential challenges. You can find plenty of resources online, including blogs, books, and documentaries that will help you make informed decisions.

3. Plan Your Meals

Planning is key to success when transitioning to a plant-based diet. Make a meal plan, and ensure it includes a variety of foods from different food groups. This will help you stay on track and avoid relying on processed foods and snacks.

4. Get Creative with Cooking

Cooking plant-based meals can be fun and exciting, especially if you are open to trying new foods and experimenting with different cooking techniques. There are plenty of plant-based recipe books and online resources with healthy and delicious meal ideas.

5. Be Mindful of Your Nutrient Intake

Plant-based diets can provide all the necessary nutrients if the diet is balanced and varied. Be mindful of nutrient intake, especially calcium, iron, vitamin B12, and omega-3 fatty acids, which can be obtained through plant-based sources such as leafy greens, nuts, and seeds.

6. Don't Be Too Hard On Yourself

Transitioning to a new diet can be challenging, and it's okay to make mistakes. Don't beat yourself up if you slip up and eat meat or dairy products. Instead, focus on making positive changes to your diet and lifestyle.

In conclusion, transitioning to a plant-based diet can be a rewarding and healthy lifestyle change that benefits your overall health and well-being. Start slowly, educate yourself, plan your meals, get creative with cooking, be mindful of nutrient intake, and don't be too hard on yourself. With time and patience, you will be able to fully embrace a plant-based lifestyle.

Plant-Based Fitness Tips

Plant-based Fitness Tips

With the growing popularity of plant-based diets, many people are now turning to this lifestyle to improve their health and fitness. Whether you are already a vegan or just starting, here are some plant-based fitness tips to help you achieve your goals:

1. Fuel your body with plant-based protein

Protein is essential for building and repairing muscle tissue, and it's important to get enough of it in your diet. Luckily, there are plenty of plant-based protein sources to choose from, such as beans, lentils, tofu, tempeh, and quinoa. Incorporate these foods into your meals to ensure you are getting enough protein to support your fitness goals.

2. Eat a variety of colorful fruits and vegetables

Fruits and vegetables are packed with essential vitamins, minerals, and antioxidants that can help you stay healthy and energized. Aim to eat a variety of colorful fruits and vegetables every day to ensure you are getting all the nutrients your body needs to perform at its best.

3. Hydrate with water and plant-based beverages

Staying hydrated is important for overall health and fitness, and it's especially important when you are active. Drink plenty of water throughout the day, and consider incorporating plant-based beverages like coconut water or herbal tea to add variety and flavor to your routine.

4. Experiment with plant-based supplements

Plant-based supplements like spirulina, chlorella, and maca powder can provide additional nutrients to support your fitness goals. Talk to your healthcare provider or a registered dietitian to determine which supplements might be right for you.

5. Incorporate mindfulness practices into your routine

Holistic practices like meditation, yoga, and tai chi can help reduce stress, improve focus, and promote overall well-being. Incorporate these practices into your fitness routine to help you stay motivated and centered.

Whether you are focused on weight loss, senior fitness, or simply staying healthy and active, these plant-based fitness tips can help you achieve your goals. Remember to listen to your body, stay consistent with your routine, and have fun along the way!

HOLISTIC NUTRITION AND FITNESS

What is holistic nutrition?

In recent years, the term "holistic nutrition" has become increasingly popular in the world of health and wellness. But what exactly does it mean?

At its core, holistic nutrition is an approach to eating that focuses on the entire person – body, mind, and spirit – rather than just individual nutrients or food groups. It emphasizes the importance of eating whole, nutrient-dense foods to support optimal health and well-being.

Unlike many traditional diets, which may focus solely on weight loss or certain health markers, holistic nutrition takes a more comprehensive view of health. It recognizes that factors such as stress, sleep, and emotional well-being can all impact our overall health and nutrition.

So, what does a holistic approach to nutrition look like in practice? Here are a few key principles:

1. Focus on whole foods: Holistic nutrition emphasizes the importance of eating whole, nutrient-dense foods such as fruits, vegetables, whole grains, and lean proteins. These foods provide a wide range of nutrients that support overall health and well-being.

2. Consider the quality of your food: Holistic nutrition also

emphasizes the importance of choosing high-quality, minimally processed foods. This means looking for foods that are organic, non-GMO, and free from artificial additives and preservatives.

3. Pay attention to how you eat: Holistic nutrition also emphasizes the importance of mindful eating. This means paying attention to your hunger and fullness cues, eating slowly and savoring your food, and avoiding distractions such as TV or work during meals.

4. Consider the bigger picture: Finally, holistic nutrition takes into account the many factors that can impact our health and nutrition. This includes stress, sleep, and emotional well-being, as well as environmental factors such as pollution and toxins.

In summary, holistic nutrition is an approach to eating that takes a comprehensive view of health and well-being. By focusing on whole, nutrient-dense foods and considering the many factors that impact our health, we can support optimal health and well-being at any age.

The Mind-Body Connection

The mind-body connection is an essential component of overall health and wellness. It is the relationship between our mental and emotional well-being and our physical health. Research has shown that our thoughts and feelings can have a significant impact on our physical health.

When we experience stress, our bodies release hormones like cortisol and adrenaline, which can affect our immune system, digestive system, and cardiovascular system. Chronic stress can lead to inflammation, which is linked to a variety of health problems, including heart disease, diabetes, and cancer.

On the other hand, positive emotions, like joy and gratitude, can have a beneficial effect on our health. They can boost the immune system, reduce inflammation, and improve cardiovascular health. Meditation, yoga, and other mindfulness practices can also have a positive impact on our physical health by reducing stress and promoting relaxation.

In addition to the impact of emotions on physical health, the mind-body connection also plays a role in our behavior and lifestyle choices. Our thoughts and beliefs can influence our motivation, self-esteem, and confidence, which can impact our ability to make healthy choices like exercising regularly and eating a nutritious diet.

For those interested in plant-based nutrition and fitness or holistic nutrition and fitness, it is important to consider the mind-body connection when making lifestyle choices. Mindful eating practices like paying attention to hunger and fullness cues and savoring food can enhance the enjoyment and satisfaction of plant-based meals. Mind-body practices like yoga and meditation can also support physical health and emotional well-being.

For those interested in weight loss nutrition and fitness, the mind-body connection can be a powerful tool in achieving and maintaining a healthy weight. Addressing emotional eating patterns and stress management can help create a sustainable weight loss plan.

For seniors and children, the mind-body connection can play a critical role in overall health and well-being. Physical activity and social engagement can improve cognitive function and reduce the risk of depression and anxiety.

Finally, for busy professionals, the mind-body connection can be a valuable tool for managing stress and maintaining work-life balance. Incorporating mindfulness practices into the workday, like taking mindful breaks or incorporating movement into the workday, can help support overall health and well-being.

In conclusion, the mind-body connection is an essential component of overall health and wellness. By understanding the relationship between our mental and emotional well-being and our physical health, we can make informed choices to support our health and well-being at any age or stage of life.

Holistic Fitness Practices

Holistic fitness practices aim to promote overall well-being and balance in the body, mind, and spirit. This approach to fitness involves combining physical exercise with mindfulness, nutrition, and self-care practices to create a comprehensive and sustainable fitness routine.

One of the key principles of holistic fitness is to focus on the quality of movement rather than just the quantity or intensity of the exercise. This means paying attention to your body's needs and limitations and choosing exercises that promote flexibility, mobility, and strength without causing pain or injury.

Another important aspect of holistic fitness is nutrition. Eating a well-balanced, plant-based diet that is rich in whole foods can provide the body with the nutrients it needs to fuel physical activity and support overall health. In addition, practicing mindfulness and stress-reduction techniques can help improve digestion, reduce inflammation, and support healthy immune function.

Holistic fitness also includes self-care practices such as massage, yoga, meditation, and other relaxation techniques. These practices can help reduce stress, improve sleep quality, and promote a sense of calm and balance in daily life.

For seniors and children, holistic fitness practices can be tailored to meet their unique needs and abilities. Older adults may benefit from low-impact exercises such as walking, swimming, and gentle yoga, while children can benefit from activities such as dance, gymnastics, and play-based exercises that promote coordination and balance.

Busy professionals can also benefit from holistic fitness practices by incorporating mindfulness techniques such as deep breathing, yoga, or meditation into their daily routines. This can help reduce stress and improve focus, leading to greater productivity and overall well-being.

In conclusion, holistic fitness practices can provide a comprehensive and sustainable approach to fitness that promotes overall health and well-being. By combining physical exercise with mindfulness, nutrition, and self-care practices, individuals of all ages and fitness levels can achieve their health goals and lead fulfilling, balanced lives.

Holistic Nutrition And Fitness Tips

Holistic Nutrition and Fitness Tips

When it comes to nutrition and fitness, many people focus solely on the physical aspects, such as weight loss or building muscle. However, a holistic approach takes into account not only the body but also the mind and spirit. Here are some tips for achieving holistic nutrition and fitness:

1. Eat whole, plant-based foods - A plant-based diet provides the nutrients and fiber your body needs to function optimally. Focus on whole foods such as fruits, vegetables, whole grains, legumes, nuts, and seeds.

2. Practice mindful eating - Eating mindfully means paying attention to your body's hunger and fullness signals, and being present in the moment while eating. This can help you avoid overeating and improve digestion.

3. Stay hydrated - Drinking enough water is crucial for maintaining good health. Aim for at least 8 glasses of water per day, and more if you are active or in hot weather.

4. Move your body - Exercise is important for maintaining physical and mental health. Find an activity that you enjoy, whether it's walking, yoga, dancing, or weight lifting. Consistency is key - aim for at least 30 minutes of moderate exercise most days of the week.

5. Practice stress management - Stress can have negative impacts on both physical and mental health. Find ways to manage stress that work for you, such as meditation, deep breathing, or spending time in nature.

6. Get enough sleep - Sleep is important for repairing and rejuvenating the body. Aim for 7-9 hours of sleep per night, and establish a consistent sleep schedule.

7. Connect with others - Social connections are crucial for mental health and well-being. Make time to connect with friends, family, or community groups.

By incorporating these holistic nutrition and fitness tips into your daily routine, you can improve your overall health and well-being. Remember that small changes over time can lead to big results and that everyone's journey is unique. Listen to your body and honor what it needs to thrive.

WEIGHT LOSS NUTRITION AND FITNESS

The basics of weight loss

The Basics of Weight Loss

Losing weight is a common goal for many people, but it can be challenging to know where to start. The key to successful weight loss is to understand the basics and make simple, sustainable changes to your lifestyle.

Calories In, Calories Out

Weight loss ultimately comes down to calories in versus calories out. To lose weight, you need to consume fewer calories than you burn each day. This can be achieved through a combination of diet and exercise.

Diet

Your diet is the foundation of your weight loss journey. To lose weight, you need to create a calorie deficit by consuming fewer calories than your body burns each day. This can be achieved by reducing portion sizes, choosing lower-calorie foods, and avoiding high-calorie, processed foods.

It's important to focus on nutrient-dense, whole foods that provide your body with the nutrients it needs to function properly. This includes plenty of fruits and vegetables, whole grains, lean proteins, and healthy fats.

Exercise

Exercise is an important component of weight loss because it helps you burn calories and build muscle. Aim for at least 150 minutes of moderate-intensity exercise per week, such as brisk walking, cycling, or swimming. You can also incorporate strength training to build muscle and boost your metabolism.

Other Strategies

In addition to diet and exercise, there are other strategies that can support weight loss. These include:

- Getting enough sleep: Lack of sleep can disrupt hormones that regulate appetite and metabolism, making it harder to lose weight.

- Managing stress: Stress can lead to overeating and poor food choices. Find healthy ways to manage stress, such as meditation or yoga.

- Drinking plenty of water: Staying hydrated can help you feel full and reduce cravings.

- Tracking your progress: Keeping track of your weight and measurements can help you stay motivated and make adjustments to your diet and exercise routine as needed.

In conclusion, weight loss is achievable for all ages and niches with a basic understanding of creating a calorie deficit through diet and exercise. Incorporating other strategies such as sleep, stress management, hydration, and tracking progress can also support successful weight loss. Remember to make sustainable changes to your lifestyle that you can maintain long-term for optimal health and wellness.

Nutrition for weight loss

Nutrition for Weight Loss

Losing weight can be a daunting task, but with the right nutrition, it can be achievable. Nutrition is the foundation of successful weight loss, and it is important to understand the relationship between food and your body's metabolism.

The first step in weight loss nutrition is to reduce your overall calorie intake. This can be done by consuming smaller portions, choosing low-calorie foods, and avoiding high-calorie snacks and drinks. It is also important to choose nutrient-dense foods that will keep you feeling full and satisfied.

Protein is a key nutrient for weight loss as it helps to build and repair muscle tissue, which can increase your metabolism. Good sources of protein include lean meats, fish, eggs, beans, and nuts. Fiber is also important for weight loss as it helps to fill you up and keeps you feeling full for longer periods of time. Foods high in fiber include whole grains, fruits, vegetables, and legumes.

Another important aspect of weight loss nutrition is hydration. Drinking plenty of water can help to flush out toxins, reduce bloating, and prevent overeating. It is recommended to drink at least eight glasses of water per day.

In addition to making healthy food choices, incorporating physical activity into your daily routine is essential for weight loss. Exercise not only burns calories but also helps to build muscle, which can increase your metabolism.

It is important to remember that weight loss is a journey, and it takes time and effort to achieve your goals. It is also important to consult with a healthcare professional before starting any weight loss program to ensure it is safe and effective for you.

In conclusion, nutrition plays a vital role in weight loss, and it is important to make healthy food choices, stay hydrated, and incorporate physical activity into your daily routine. By following these guidelines and seeking professional guidance, you can achieve a healthy weight and improve your overall well-being.

Fitness For Weight Loss

Fitness for Weight Loss

Weight loss is a common goal for many people, and achieving it requires a combination of healthy eating and regular exercise. Exercise is not only essential for burning calories but also for building muscle, boosting metabolism, and improving overall health.

When it comes to weight loss, there are many types of exercises you can do. However, the most effective ones are those that get your heart rate up and keep it elevated for an extended period. These include cardio exercises such as running, cycling, swimming, dancing, and high-intensity interval training (HIIT).

Incorporating resistance training into your workout routine is also crucial for weight loss. It helps to build lean muscle mass, which in turn burns more calories even at rest. Resistance training can be done using weights, resistance bands, or bodyweight exercises such as push-ups, squats, and lunges.

It is essential to remember that weight loss is not just about exercising. It also requires a healthy and balanced diet. Eating a diet rich in whole foods such as fruits, vegetables, whole grains, and lean proteins is key. Avoiding processed and high-fat foods is also crucial.

In addition to exercise and a healthy diet, staying hydrated is also essential for weight loss. Drinking plenty of water helps to boost metabolism, flush out toxins, and reduce hunger cravings.

For those looking to lose weight, it is essential to keep in mind that it is a journey and not a quick fix. It requires patience, dedication, and consistency. It is also crucial to listen to your body and work within your limits. Gradual progress is better than quick results that are not sustainable.

In conclusion, fitness plays a crucial role in weight loss. Incorporating a combination of cardio, resistance training, and a healthy diet is the most effective way to achieve your weight loss goals. Remember to stay hydrated, listen to your body, and be patient with the process.

Weight Loss Tips And Tricks

Weight Loss Tips and Tricks

Losing weight can be a daunting task for many people, but it doesn't have to be. With some simple changes to your diet and lifestyle, you can achieve your weight loss goals and improve your overall health and well-being.

1. Eat more whole foods: One of the best things you can do for your health and weight loss is to eat more whole foods. These are foods that are minimally processed and contain all the nutrients your body needs. Whole foods include fruits, vegetables, whole grains, lean proteins, and healthy fats.

2. Cut out processed foods: Processed foods are often high in calories, unhealthy fats, and sugar. By cutting out these foods, you can reduce your calorie intake and improve your overall health. Instead, opt for whole foods and cook your meals at home whenever possible.

3. Drink more water: Drinking water can help you lose weight by reducing your appetite and increasing your metabolism. Aim for at least eight glasses of water a day, and avoid sugary drinks like soda and juice.

4. Get enough sleep: Lack of sleep can lead to weight gain and other health problems. Aim for at least seven hours of sleep a night, and try to establish a regular sleep schedule.

5. Exercise regularly: Exercise is crucial for weight loss and overall health. Aim for at least 30 minutes of moderate-intensity exercise most days of the week. You can also incorporate strength training

to build muscle and boost your metabolism.

6. Practice mindful eating: Mindful eating involves paying attention to your body's hunger and fullness cues and eating slowly and without distractions. This can help you eat less and enjoy your food more.

7. Keep a food diary: Keeping track of what you eat can help you stay accountable and identify areas where you can make healthier choices. Use a food diary or app to track your meals and snacks.

8. Find support: Losing weight can be challenging, but having support can make a big difference. Join a support group or find a friend or family member who can support and encourage you on your weight loss journey.

By incorporating these tips and tricks into your daily routine, you can achieve your weight loss goals and improve your overall health and well-being. Remember to be patient and consistent, and celebrate your progress along the way.

NUTRITION AND FITNESS FOR SENIORS

The importance of nutrition and fitness for seniors

The importance of nutrition and fitness for seniors cannot be overstated. As we age, our bodies change and require different nutrients and exercise routines to maintain optimal health. Proper nutrition and fitness can help seniors maintain their independence, prevent chronic diseases, and improve their overall quality of life.

Nutrition is an essential aspect of healthy aging, and seniors need to pay close attention to what they eat. Eating a balanced diet with plenty of fruits, vegetables, whole grains, lean protein, and healthy fats can help seniors maintain a healthy weight, boost their immune system, and reduce their risk of chronic diseases such as diabetes, heart disease, and cancer.

In addition to eating a balanced diet, seniors should also make sure they are getting enough calcium and vitamin D to maintain strong bones and prevent osteoporosis. They should also stay hydrated by drinking plenty of water and limiting their intake of sugary drinks.

Exercise is also crucial for seniors, as it can help maintain muscle mass, improve balance and flexibility, and reduce the risk of falls. Seniors should aim for at least 150 minutes of moderate-intensity exercise per week, which can include activities such as brisk walking, swimming, or cycling.

It's never too late to start exercising, and seniors should consult their doctor before starting any new exercise routine. They should also choose activities that they enjoy and that are appropriate for their fitness level.

In addition to nutrition and exercise, seniors should also prioritize getting enough sleep and managing stress. Poor sleep habits and chronic stress can have negative effects on overall health and well-being.

In conclusion, nutrition and fitness are crucial for seniors to maintain their health and independence. By eating a balanced diet, staying hydrated, getting enough exercise, and prioritizing sleep and stress management, seniors can improve their overall quality of life and reduce their risk of chronic diseases.

Senior-specific nutrition needs

Senior-specific nutrition needs

As we age, our bodies undergo a variety of changes that can affect our nutritional needs. Some of these changes include a decrease in muscle mass, a decrease in bone density, and changes in our digestive system. Seniors need to pay close attention to their nutrition to maintain good health and prevent age-related diseases.

One of the most important nutrients for seniors is protein. As we age, our bodies become less efficient at using protein to build and repair muscle tissue. This can lead to a loss of muscle mass and strength, which can increase the risk of falls and other injuries. Seniors should aim to consume at least 1.2 grams of protein per kilogram of body weight per day. Good sources of protein include lean meats, fish, poultry, eggs, beans, and nuts.

Another important nutrient for seniors is calcium. As we age, our bones become more brittle and are more prone to fractures. Calcium is essential for maintaining strong bones and teeth. Seniors should aim to consume at least 1,200 milligrams of calcium per day. Good sources of calcium include dairy products, leafy green vegetables, and fortified foods such as cereal and orange juice.

In addition to protein and calcium, seniors should also pay attention to their intake of vitamins and minerals. Some vitamins and minerals that are especially important for seniors include vitamin D, vitamin B12, and potassium. Vitamin D is important for maintaining strong bones and may also help prevent certain diseases such as cancer and diabetes. Seniors should aim to get at least 600-800 IU of vitamin D per day. Good sources of vitamin D include sunlight, fatty fish, and fortified foods such as milk and cereal.

Vitamin B12 is important for maintaining healthy nerve cells and red blood cells. As we age, our bodies become less efficient at absorbing vitamin B12 from food. Seniors should aim to consume at least 2.4 micrograms of vitamin B12 per day. Good sources of vitamin B12 include meat, fish, poultry, and fortified foods such as cereal.

Potassium is important for maintaining healthy blood pressure and may also help prevent certain diseases such as stroke and heart disease. Seniors should aim to consume at least 4,700 milligrams of potassium per day. Good sources of potassium include bananas, potatoes, tomatoes, and leafy green vegetables.

In conclusion, seniors have specific nutritional needs that must be met to maintain good health and prevent age-related diseases. A diet that is high in protein, calcium, vitamins, and minerals is essential for seniors. By focusing on these key nutrients, seniors can enjoy a healthy and active lifestyle well into their golden years.

Senior-Specific Fitness Tips

Senior-specific fitness tips

As we age, it becomes more important than ever to maintain

an active lifestyle. Exercise helps to reduce the risk of chronic diseases, improves mobility and balance, and can even enhance cognitive function. Here are some senior-specific fitness tips to help you stay healthy and active.

1. Focus on strength training

Strength training is crucial for seniors as it helps to maintain muscle mass and bone density. Aim to do strength training exercises at least twice a week, focusing on major muscle groups such as the legs, arms, back, and chest. You can use weights, resistance bands, or your body weight to perform exercises such as squats, lunges, push-ups, and tricep dips.

2. Prioritize balance and flexibility

As we age, our balance and flexibility can decline, making us more prone to falls and injuries. Incorporate balance and flexibility exercises into your routine, such as yoga, tai chi, or simple balance exercises like standing on one leg. These exercises can help to improve your balance and reduce the risk of falls.

3. Mix up your cardio

Cardiovascular exercise is important for heart health and overall fitness, but it's important to mix up your activities to avoid boredom and reduce the risk of injury. Try activities like walking, swimming, cycling, or dancing to get your heart rate up and improve your endurance.

4. Listen to your body

As we age, it's important to listen to our bodies and not push ourselves too hard. If a particular exercise or activity causes pain or discomfort, modify or skip it altogether. Be sure to warm up properly before exercising and cool down afterward to prevent injury.

5. Stay hydrated

Dehydration can be a serious issue for seniors, so it's important to drink plenty of water throughout the day. Aim for at least eight glasses of water per day, and more if you're exercising or in hot weather.

Incorporating these senior-specific fitness tips into your routine can help you stay healthy and active as you age. Remember, it's never too late to start exercising and reaping the benefits of a healthy lifestyle.

Senior-specific nutrition and fitness challenges

As we age, our bodies change and require different nutritional and fitness needs. Seniors face unique challenges when it comes to maintaining their health and wellness. It's important to understand these challenges and work towards a healthy lifestyle to prevent or manage age-related health problems.

One of the challenges seniors face is a decrease in appetite. This can be due to a variety of factors such as a decrease in taste and smell, medications, or health conditions. Seniors need to eat nutrient-dense foods to meet their nutritional needs. This means incorporating plenty of fruits, vegetables, whole grains, and lean protein into their diet.

Another challenge seniors face is a decrease in muscle mass and bone density. This can lead to an increased risk of falls and fractures. Incorporating strength training exercises into their fitness routine can help increase muscle mass and bone density. Seniors need to consult with a doctor or certified personal trainer before starting a new exercise routine.

Seniors may also face dental problems, making it difficult to chew and swallow certain foods. Incorporating smoothies and soups into their diet can help ensure they are getting the necessary nutrients.

Dehydration is another common problem among seniors. They may not feel thirsty or may forget to drink water throughout the day. Seniors need to drink plenty of fluids, especially water, to prevent dehydration.

Finally, seniors may face social isolation, which can lead to depression and other health problems. Participating in group fitness classes or social activities can help seniors stay connected and improve their overall well-being.

In conclusion, seniors face unique challenges when it comes to nutrition and fitness. They need to eat nutrient-dense foods, incorporate strength training exercises, stay hydrated, and participate in social activities to maintain their health and wellness. By understanding these challenges and working towards a healthy lifestyle, seniors can prevent or manage age-related health problems and live fulfilling lives.

NUTRITION AND FITNESS FOR CHILDREN

The importance of nutrition and fitness for children

The health of children is of utmost importance, and nutrition and fitness play a crucial role in maintaining their overall well-being. A healthy diet and regular exercise can help children develop physically, mentally, and emotionally, paving the way for a healthy future. Here are some reasons why nutrition and fitness are so important for children:

1. Physical Development: A healthy diet and regular exercise help children develop strong bones, muscles, and organs, which are essential for growth and development. Proper nutrition ensures that children get all the nutrients they need for healthy growth, while exercise helps build strong muscles and bones.

2. Mental Health: Good nutrition and exercise are also essential for mental health. A balanced diet can help improve mood and cognitive function, while regular exercise can reduce stress and anxiety.

3. Disease Prevention: A healthy diet and regular exercise can also help prevent chronic diseases such as obesity, diabetes, and heart disease. By encouraging children to eat a variety of fruits,

vegetables, whole grains, and lean proteins, parents can help reduce their risk of developing these conditions later in life.

4. Energy: Proper nutrition and exercise can also help children maintain energy levels throughout the day. A balanced diet provides the nutrients needed for sustained energy, while exercise helps stimulate the production of endorphins, which can boost mood and energy levels.

5. Self-Esteem: Good nutrition and exercise can also help improve a child's self-esteem. By encouraging healthy habits, parents can help children feel good about themselves and their bodies, which can lead to improved self-confidence and self-worth.

In conclusion, nutrition and fitness are crucial for the health and well-being of children. By instilling healthy habits early on, parents can help children develop into healthy, happy adults. Whether your child is a picky eater or a budding athlete, there are many ways to encourage healthy habits and set them up for a lifetime of good health.

Children's Nutrition Needs

Children's Nutrition Needs

As parents, caregivers, or guardians, we all want our children to grow up healthy and strong. One of the most important ways to achieve this is through proper nutrition. Children have unique nutritional needs that vary depending on their age, gender, activity level, and overall health status.

Infants and toddlers require more fat and calories than older children and adults to support their rapid growth and development. Breast milk or formula provides the necessary nutrients for infants up to six months old. After that, solid foods can be introduced gradually, starting with iron-fortified cereals, pureed fruits and vegetables, and mashed proteins such as eggs, tofu, or well-cooked meat.

Preschoolers and school-aged children need a balanced diet that includes carbohydrates, protein, healthy fats, vitamins, and minerals. They also need more calcium and vitamin D for their growing bones and teeth. Offer them a variety of colorful fruits and vegetables, whole grains, lean meats, fish, legumes, nuts, and seeds. Limit their intake of processed and sugary foods and beverages, such as soda, candy, cookies, and chips.

It's also essential to encourage children to drink plenty of water throughout the day, especially when they are active or in hot weather. Milk and 100% fruit juice can be consumed in moderation, but be aware of their added sugar and calorie content. Avoid giving children energy drinks, sports drinks, or caffeinated beverages, as they can have adverse effects on their health and behavior.

If you have a picky eater or a child with a food allergy or intolerance, consult with a registered dietitian or pediatrician to ensure that their nutritional needs are met. Don't force them to eat or restrict certain foods, as this can create negative associations with food and lead to disordered eating habits.

In summary, children's nutrition needs are crucial for their growth, development, and overall health. Offer them a balanced and varied diet, encourage them to drink water, and seek professional help if needed. By instilling healthy eating habits in children, you can set them up for a lifetime of wellness and happiness.

Children's Fitness Tips

Children's Fitness Tips

Ensuring that children stay active and healthy is crucial for their overall well-being. In today's world, with the rise of technology and sedentary activities, it can be challenging to encourage children to engage in physical activities. In this subchapter, we will explore some tips to help children stay active and healthy.

1. Make it fun

Children love to have fun, and physical activities should be no different. Engage in activities that your child enjoys, such as dancing, swimming, or playing sports. You can also make it a family affair by going for hikes, bike rides, or playing in the park together.

2. Encourage outdoor play

Outdoor play can offer a multitude of benefits for children. It can help improve their physical fitness, promote social skills, and reduce stress levels. Encourage your child to engage in outdoor activities, such as playing in the park, riding their bike or scooter, or going for a nature walk.

3. Limit screen time

Excessive screen time can have detrimental effects on a child's health. Limit the amount of time your child spends in front of screens, including TVs, computers, and mobile devices. Encourage them to engage in physical activities or other hobbies that do not involve screen time.

4. Make physical activity a part of the daily routine

Incorporating physical activity into a child's daily routine can help establish healthy habits. Encourage your child to engage in physical activities, such as walking or biking to school or participating in sports teams.

5. Provide healthy snacks and meals

Nutrition plays a crucial role in a child's overall health and fitness. Provide your child with healthy snacks and meals that are rich in nutrients, such as fruits, vegetables, whole grains, and lean proteins.

In conclusion, ensuring that children stay active and healthy is essential for their overall well-being. By making physical activity fun, encouraging outdoor play, limiting screen time, making physical activity a part of the daily routine, and providing healthy snacks and meals, you can help your child establish healthy habits that will benefit them for a lifetime.

Children's Nutrition And Fitness Challenges

Children's nutrition and fitness challenges are a growing concern in today's society. With the rise of technology and busy schedules, it can be difficult for children to get the proper nutrition and exercise they need to stay healthy. There are several challenges that children face when it comes to their nutrition and fitness, and parents and caregivers need to be aware of these challenges and take steps to overcome them.

One of the biggest challenges facing children today is the prevalence of processed and fast foods. These foods are often high in calories, fat, and sugar, and lack the nutrients that children need to grow and develop properly. Additionally, many children are not getting enough physical activity, which can lead to obesity and other health problems.

Another challenge is the increasingly sedentary lifestyle of children. With the rise of technology, many children spend hours each day sitting in front of screens, whether it's watching TV, playing video games, or using their smartphones or tablets. This lack of physical activity can harm their health and well-being.

Parents and caregivers can help children overcome these challenges by encouraging healthy eating habits and regular physical activity. This can include providing healthy meals and snacks, limiting processed and fast foods, and encouraging children to participate in physical activities they enjoy, such as sports, dance, or martial arts.

It's also important to teach children about the importance of nutrition and fitness and to lead by example. Parents and caregivers can set a good example by eating healthy foods, exercising regularly, and making health a priority in their own lives.

In conclusion, children's nutrition and fitness challenges are a growing concern, but there are steps that parents and caregivers can take to help children overcome these challenges. By providing healthy meals and snacks, encouraging physical activity, and teaching children about the importance of nutrition and fitness, we can help children lead healthy, active lives.

NUTRITION AND FITNESS FOR BUSY PROFESSIONALS

The challenges of maintaining a healthy lifestyle while working

The Challenges of Maintaining a Healthy Lifestyle while Working

In today's fast-paced world, it can be challenging to maintain a healthy lifestyle while working. This is especially true for those who work long hours or have demanding jobs. However, it is essential to prioritize your health and take care of your body and mind to achieve optimal performance at work and in life. In this chapter, we will explore some of the challenges of maintaining a healthy lifestyle while working and provide practical solutions to overcome them.

One of the biggest challenges of maintaining a healthy lifestyle while working is finding the time to exercise. Many people struggle to fit regular exercise into their busy schedules, leading to a sedentary lifestyle and associated health problems. However, there are many ways to incorporate physical activity into your workday, such as taking short walks during breaks or using a standing desk. You can also join a gym near your office, take fitness classes during lunch breaks, or find a workout buddy to keep you motivated.

Another challenge is eating healthy while working. Many people rely on fast food or vending machines for their meals, which can lead to weight gain and other health issues. To overcome this challenge, you can plan your meals, pack healthy snacks and lunches, and avoid sugary drinks and processed foods. You can also opt for plant-based nutrition and fitness, which offers a range of health benefits and can be easily incorporated into your work routine.

Moreover, stress is another factor that can impact your health while working. High levels of stress can lead to burnout, anxiety, depression, and other health problems. To manage stress, you can practice mindfulness, meditation, yoga, or other relaxation techniques. You can also take regular breaks, prioritize self-care, and seek support from friends, family, or a professional therapist.

In conclusion, maintaining a healthy lifestyle while working can be challenging, but it is essential for your overall well-being and success. By incorporating physical activity, healthy eating habits, stress management techniques, and self-care into your work routine, you can achieve optimal health and performance in all areas of your life.

Nutrition Tips For Busy Professionals

Nutrition tips for busy professionals

In today's fast-paced world, it's easy to fall into the trap of prioritizing work over health. However, neglecting your nutrition and fitness can lead to a variety of health problems, including obesity, heart disease, and diabetes. As a busy professional, it's important to make time for your health. Here are some nutrition tips that can help you stay on track:

1. Plan ahead

One of the biggest obstacles to eating healthy is lack of time. To overcome this, take some time each week to plan your meals. This will help you avoid impulsive food choices and ensure that you have healthy options available when you're short on time.

2. Make healthy swaps

Small changes can make a big difference in your overall health. Swap out unhealthy snacks like chips and candy for healthier options like fruit, nuts, and seeds. Choose whole-grain bread over white bread, and opt for lean protein sources like chicken and fish instead of red meat.

3. Keep healthy snacks on hand

When you're working long hours, it's easy to reach for a bag of chips or a candy bar. To avoid this temptation, keep healthy snacks on hand at all times. This could include fruits, vegetables, nuts, and seeds.

4. Don't skip meals

Skipping meals can lead to overeating later on, as well as a drop in energy levels. Even if you're short on time, make sure to have a healthy breakfast, lunch, and dinner. If you're really pressed for time, try meal prepping on the weekends so you have healthy meals ready to go throughout the week.

5. Stay hydrated

Drinking enough water is crucial for good health. Aim to drink at least eight glasses of water a day, and avoid sugary drinks like soda and juice.

6. Take breaks

Sitting for long periods of time can be detrimental to your health. Take breaks throughout the day to stretch, walk around, and get some fresh air. This will help you stay energized and focused throughout the day.

By following these nutrition tips, you can prioritize your health and fitness even when you're busy. Remember, your health is your most important asset, so make sure to take care of it!

Fitness Tips For Busy Professionals

Fitness Tips for Busy Professionals

Being a busy professional can make it challenging to maintain a healthy and active lifestyle. It's easy to get caught up in the daily grind and forget that our health should always be a top priority. However, with a few simple tweaks to your routine, you can make fitness a part of your daily life. Here are some fitness tips for busy professionals:

1. Schedule Your Workouts

One of the most effective ways to ensure that you get your workouts in is to schedule them into your calendar. Treat your workouts like any other important appointment and don't cancel them. You'll be more likely to stick to your fitness routine if you make it a priority.

2. Plan Ahead

Meal planning and preparation can save you time and ensure that you're eating healthy meals throughout the week. Spend a few hours on the weekend prepping your meals for the week ahead. This will help you avoid the temptation of grabbing fast food or unhealthy snacks when you're busy.

3. Make the Most of Your Time

If you only have a short amount of time to work out, make the most of it. High-intensity interval training (HIIT) is a great way to get a full-body workout in a short amount of time. You can also try incorporating exercise into your daily routine, such as taking the stairs instead of the elevator or going for a walk during your lunch break.

4. Stay Hydrated

Drinking enough water is essential for staying healthy and energized throughout the day. Keep a water bottle with you at all times and aim to drink at least eight glasses of water per day. You can also add fresh fruit or herbs to your water for some extra flavor.

5. Get Enough Sleep

Sleep is essential for overall health and well-being. Aim to get at least seven to eight hours of sleep per night. If you're having trouble sleeping, try establishing a bedtime routine, avoiding electronics before bed, and creating a comfortable sleep environment.

In conclusion, being a busy professional doesn't mean you have to sacrifice your health and fitness. By scheduling your workouts, planning, making the most of your time, staying hydrated, and getting enough sleep, you can maintain a healthy and active lifestyle. Remember, your health should always be a top priority.

Strategies For Making Healthy Choices On-The-Go

In our fast-paced world, it can be challenging to make healthy choices on the go. Whether you are a busy professional, a senior, or a parent with young children, it is important to prioritize your health and make good choices when you are out and about.

One strategy for making healthy choices on the go is to plan. Take a few minutes to pack healthy snacks and meals to bring with you when you leave the house. This can include fresh fruit, nuts, and seeds, cut-up veggies, and pre-made salads or sandwiches.

Another strategy is to choose healthy options when you are eating out. Look for restaurants that offer healthy options on their menus or ask for modifications to your meal to make them healthier. Avoid fried and processed foods and choose dishes that are baked, grilled, or steamed.

If you are in a rush and need to grab something quickly, look for healthy grab-and-go options. Many convenience stores and gas stations now offer healthy snacks like fresh fruit, trail mix, and protein bars. You can also find pre-packaged salads, sandwiches, and wraps at many supermarkets.

Staying hydrated is also important when you are on the go. Carry a reusable water bottle with you and refill it throughout the day. Avoid sugary drinks like soda and juice and opt for water, herbal tea, or unsweetened iced tea instead.

If you are traveling, it can be especially challenging to make healthy choices. Plan by packing healthy snacks and researching restaurants that offer healthy options. You can also bring along a small cooler with pre-made meals and snacks.

Overall, making healthy choices on the go requires a bit of planning and preparation. But by prioritizing your health and making good choices, you can stay on track with your nutrition and fitness goals no matter where life takes you.

Conclusion

The importance of maintaining a healthy lifestyle

Maintaining a healthy lifestyle is crucial for a happy and fulfilling life. It is essential to understand that good health is not just about being free from illnesses but also about having a positive and energetic outlook on life. In this chapter, we will discuss the importance of maintaining a healthy lifestyle and how it can benefit people of all ages.

Nutrition and Fitness

A healthy lifestyle includes a balanced diet and regular physical activity. A balanced diet is essential for providing the body with the necessary nutrients to function optimally. Regular physical activity is crucial for maintaining a healthy weight, building strength, and reducing the risk of chronic diseases.

Plant-based Nutrition and Fitness

Plant-based nutrition and fitness are gaining popularity due to their numerous health benefits. A plant-based diet is rich in fiber, vitamins, and minerals, which can help reduce the risk of chronic diseases such as heart disease, diabetes, and cancer. Regular physical activity can also help improve cardiovascular health, build strength, and improve overall health and well-being.

Holistic Nutrition and Fitness

Holistic nutrition and fitness focus on the mind-body connection and aim to improve overall health and well-being. A holistic approach includes nourishing the body with whole, nutrient-dense foods, and regular physical activity. In addition, stress reduction techniques such as meditation, yoga, and deep breathing can also help improve overall health and well-being.

Weight Loss Nutrition and Fitness

Maintaining a healthy weight is essential for reducing the risk of chronic diseases such as heart disease, diabetes, and cancer. A healthy weight can be achieved through a combination of a balanced diet and regular physical activity. It is important to adopt a sustainable approach to weight loss that includes making healthy lifestyle choices and not just focusing on short-term results.

Nutrition and Fitness for Seniors

As people age, the body undergoes several changes that can affect overall health and well-being. A healthy lifestyle that includes a balanced diet and regular physical activity can help reduce the risk of chronic diseases, improve cognitive function, and maintain independence and mobility.

Nutrition and Fitness for Children

Children require adequate nutrition and regular physical activity for healthy growth and development. A balanced diet that includes a variety of fruits, vegetables, whole grains, and lean protein, along with regular physical activity, is essential for optimal health and well-being.

Nutrition and Fitness for Busy Professionals

Maintaining a healthy lifestyle can be challenging for busy professionals. However, it is essential to prioritize health and make time for a balanced diet and regular physical activity. Making small, sustainable changes to daily routines can help improve overall health and well-being, reduce stress, and increase productivity.

In conclusion, maintaining a healthy lifestyle is essential for overall health and well-being. A balanced diet and regular physical activity can help reduce the risk of chronic diseases, improve cognitive function, and increase energy levels. Adopting a sustainable approach to healthy living can benefit people of all ages and niches of nutrition and fitness.